Greice Brito Bitencourt

Adolescent Oral Health

Greice Brito Bitencourt

Adolescent Oral Health

Adolescents' self-perception of their oral health, their worries and fears

ScienciaScripts

Imprint

Any brand names and product names mentioned in this book are subject to trademark, brand or patent protection and are trademarks or registered trademarks of their respective holders. The use of brand names, product names, common names, trade names, product descriptions etc. even without a particular marking in this work is in no way to be construed to mean that such names may be regarded as unrestricted in respect of trademark and brand protection legislation and could thus be used by anyone.

Cover image: www.ingimage.com

This book is a translation from the original published under ISBN 978-613-9-62471-3.

Publisher:
Sciencia Scripts
is a trademark of
Dodo Books Indian Ocean Ltd. and OmniScriptum S.R.L publishing group

120 High Road, East Finchley, London, N2 9ED, United Kingdom
Str. Armeneasca 28/1, office 1, Chisinau MD-2012, Republic of Moldova, Europe
Printed at: see last page
ISBN: 978-620-7-72770-4

Summary

Dedication

I dedicate this work to my husband, who was always by my side, helping me and accepting my lack of time. My companion for so many moments, thank you for everything.

To my dear mother who has always been my safe haven, who taught me to persevere and insist on my dreams. This great woman who, even in the most difficult times, looked at me with tenderness and showed me the positive side of life.

To my father, who taught me the value of things and simplicity. The most faithful and correct friend I could ever have. I am his proudest daughter. Thank you for the years you dedicated to me.

To my siblings (Karina, Felipe and Henrique) who accepted my absence from home and who always supported me on the paths I chose to follow. Especially my younger brother, who helped me, listened to me and put up with me over the last two years. I love you all too much.

To my nephews and brother-in-law who always encouraged me and made me smile even when I was very stressed.

Thanks

To Prof. Simone Renno Junqueira, my advisor, who has accompanied and guided me since my first scientific initiation. Confident, dedicated and always a great friend. I thank her for her time and trust in me.

To my postgraduate colleagues and friends Talita Carnaval and Gisele Ebling, who have always been by my side since graduation. And they helped me with the subjects I took.

To Professor Toninho, who always had a smile on his face and helped me with this work, helping me when I was lost in the department.

To Professor Maria Ercilia, who helped me not to give up at university and always encouraged me to do my master's degree. Thank you, Professor.

To Professor Botazzo and Imparato who encouraged me to improve and gave me tips on this work.

To the secretaries of the social dentistry department who were dedicated and present during these years of study.

To the professors of the social dentistry department who always welcomed me and treated me well.

To the adolescents of Barueri who agreed to take part in this work and made it possible for this dream to come true. Summary

It is accepted that the use of health services, including dental services, should be considered in three dimensions: training, predisposition and need. This project aims to verify the training, predisposition and oral health needs of adolescents in the municipality of Barueri, in Greater São Paulo. Believing that needs go beyond those confirmed by the presence of oral diseases at the time of the epidemiological examination, we are looking for perceptions of satisfaction with the lives, bodies and oral health of these young people.

Keywords: adolescents, oral health education, predisposition, need.

1. Introduction

Universality of access to health actions and services for the promotion, protection and recovery of health is one of the principles of the Unified Health System, established by the Brazilian Constitution of 1988 (Brasil, 1988).

Brazilian public policy managers have the challenge of fulfilling this premise by developing actions that improve people's quality of life.

Oral health is also part of this context and it is hoped that universal access will lead to greater coverage of dental services.

It is believed that the expansion of coverage should be based on the epidemiological needs of the population and, to this end, epidemiological surveys in oral health have been carried out, as they make it possible to outline the profile and trend of oral diseases. More than that, they guide the planning and organization of oral health services so that they are better targeted according to needs, in accordance with the principles of equity and comprehensiveness of the Unified Health System.

The units providing services, with their varying degrees of complexity, form an indivisible whole, configuring a system capable of providing comprehensive care to the indivisible individual who is part of a community (Brazil, 1990).

Producing or maintaining a "whole man" is a task that goes far beyond the possibilities of the health services production apparatus. Rather, it is something that falls within the realm of utopia. Even with this enormous restriction, for many people a more "integralizing" approach is desirable and possible when it comes to providing health care for individuals or groups (Botazzo, 2008).

It is accepted that the use of health services, including dental services, should be considered in three dimensions: capacity, predisposition and need, as proposed by Andersen and Newman (1973). The first refers to the fact that the individual seeks and receives care, with the variables, among others, being economic conditions and the supply of services; predisposition is related to individual characteristics that increase the chances of seeking services, such as age and harmful habits; and need refers to the individual's perception of their state of health and the health condition itself, measured by its opposite, i.e. disease.

Adolescents are the target population for this study, as they have unique characteristics and attitudes, equally distinct needs and are a population group not served by preventive dental programs (Souza et al., 2007; Junqueira, 2007).

Adolescence is considered a transitional phase between childhood and youth. It is the period of life between 10 and 20 years of age, in which the young person is surprised by numerous physical, cognitive, emotional and social changes.

It is common for adolescents to behave negligently when it comes to taking care of their health. Therefore, this period is considered to be at increased risk of dental caries and other oral diseases, due to poor plaque control and less careful brushing (Who, 1995; Tomita et al., 2001).

Santos et al. (1992) agree that it is essential to know the needs and psychosocial structure of the community in which these adolescents live, incorporating them into the education program; in this way, new ideas and actions adjust, emerge and grow in this reality.

2. Justification

This project aims to verify the training, predisposition and oral health needs of adolescents in the municipality of Barueri, in Greater Sao Paulo. Believing that the needs go beyond those confirmed by the presence of oral diseases at the time of the epidemiological examination, we are looking for perceptions of satisfaction with life, body and oral health of these young people.

3. Material and Methods

3.1. Stages of the study

Using secondary data (sources: DATASUS, IBGE, SEADE, municipal oral health coordination), the offer of municipal dental services for the municipalities of Barueri is described, according to the following variables: number of oral health professionals, hours worked, number of pieces of equipment and procedures performed *(what is offered)*.

Based on the oral health epidemiological survey carried out in the municipality of Barueri in 2009, the aim is to analyze the need for dental treatment according to the following variables: need for caries treatment, need for periodontal treatment, need for dental prostheses (what is *needed)*.

In order to find out how satisfied these young people are with their lives, their bodies and their oral health, we intend to listen to the population about the social demand for oral health services (what *they ask for), using* qualitative research (Minayo, 1998).

3.2. Qualitative methodology

Qualitative research is proposed using the content analysis proposed by Bardin (1977), where, by interpreting the content of recorded interviews, units of meaning/key expressions are identified. The organization and aggregation of these units is called categorization.

The qualitative study was chosen because it deals with something little known, such as the behavior and universe of adolescents, and here we intend to describe the facts from the point of view of the subjects of the study.

Content analysis has been around since humanity's first attempts to interpret ancient writings, such as the attempts to interpret sacred books. However, it wasn't until the 1920s that content analysis was systematized as a method, due to Leavell's studies on the propaganda used in the First World War, thus acquiring the character of a research method (Trivinos, 1987).

Any communication that links a set of meanings from a sender to a receiver can, in principle, be translated by content analysis techniques.

The method of content analysis appears as a tool for understanding the construction of meaning that social actors externalize in their discourse. It is analyzed in this study from the perspective of the theory of Social Representations and the theory of Action from a phenomenological perspective. This allows the researcher to understand the representations that individuals present in relation to their reality and their interpretation of the meanings around them.

The process described refers to an interpretative view of reality from the point of view of the interviewees. This process has predominated in qualitative research, whether based on the criteria of the theory of social representations or the theory of action. These theories seek to understand reality from the interviewees' point of view, based on the discourse they declare.

Content analysis makes it possible to recognize ideas that fall into certain categories, previously identified by the researchers, and which reflect, after thorough and exhaustive analysis of the material, the thoughts, representations, beliefs and values of the research subjects on the proposed themes.

The use of content analysis takes place in three fundamental phases: pre-analysis, exploration of the material and treatment of the results.

Pre-analysis: organizing the material, all the materials that will be used for data collection, as well as materials that can help to better understand the phenomenon of adolescence.

Exploration is the phase in which you have already gathered the material that will make up the body of the research and you begin to delve deeper, being guided in principle by the hypotheses and the theoretical framework, and from this analysis tables of references emerge, looking for coinciding and diverging syntheses of ideas.

Processing the results is the phase in which you will reflect, use intuition based on empirical material, uncover the latent content, revealing ideologies and tendencies.

3.3. Data collection

To collect the material, we opted for focus group interviews. The focus group is made up of small groups of people gathered in a pre-selected location and guided by a guide drawn up by the moderator, without necessarily being limited or bound by it. Its main objective is to identify the participants' feelings, perceptions, attitudes and ideas on a given subject.

Two groups were formed, divided into male and female. The interviews were conducted using the focus group technique in December 2010 and lasted two hours for each group.

3.4. Study population

The female group had 12 girls aged 14-15 and the male group had 9 boys aged 14-17. The adolescents were in their first year of secondary school at a municipal public school in Barueri (EMF Mario Joaquim Escobar de Andrade), and the students were chosen at random by the school coordinators.

The interviews were carried out in the school itself. We set up a circle which facilitated body and visual communication.

After the introductions, the moderator started a conversation, which focused on Foucault's axes, the three major instances that Foucault distinguishes successively (Knowledge, Power and Subjectivity) do not have definitive outlines; rather, they are chains of variables related to each other.

It is always through a crisis that Foucault discovers a new dimension, a new line. Discussing themes related to work, food, body care, sex and hygiene. An assistant helped with note-taking and the perception of body language.

3.5. Research procedures and ethical aspects

The procedures adopted to carry out this research included:

- Approval report from the FOUSP Research Ethics Committee (Protocol 93/2009). (Annex C)

- A letter of request to the board of directors of the aforementioned institution to carry out the research project (Annex B).

- Requesting the signature of the person responsible for the research subject on the Free and Informed Consent form (Appendix D)

Data collection began after approval from the Ethics and Research Committee (CEP) of the University of São Paulo School of Dentistry (FOUSP), which authorized the research by sending a letter to the researcher (Appendix C).

The objectives of the study were explained to the participants. They were informed that the conversation would be recorded, but that they would not be identified, and that the conversation would last approximately two hours.

Permission was sought to record and film the conversation. This material was later transcribed in full without correcting any errors, but any information that could identify the subject was replaced by codes in the transcription.

The participants in the conversation were informed that the material analyzed will be published in scientific journals, always with the commitment not to identify them.

Research subjects were guaranteed the right to withdraw their consent at any time during the study.

4. Results and discussion

For a better understanding and discussion of the data obtained, we'll talk a little about the services offered by the municipality of Barueri (training), the data obtained in the epidemiological survey (predisposition) and the perception of these young people (needs).

4.1. Barueri Municipal Data

The municipality of Barueri has an area of 64 square kilometers and an estimated population of 273,713 inhabitants in 2008, giving a ratio of 3,509 inhabitants per km² .

Children under 15 make up 28.3% of the population and 5.65% are over 60.

The municipality has no rural areas, with the entire population concentrated in the urban area, which has 99.9% of its public roads paved (Seade, 2009).

The city is one of the main financial centers in the state of São Paulo and is the 9th richest city in Brazil.

GRAPH 1 - Demographic evolution

Demographic development of the city of Barueri

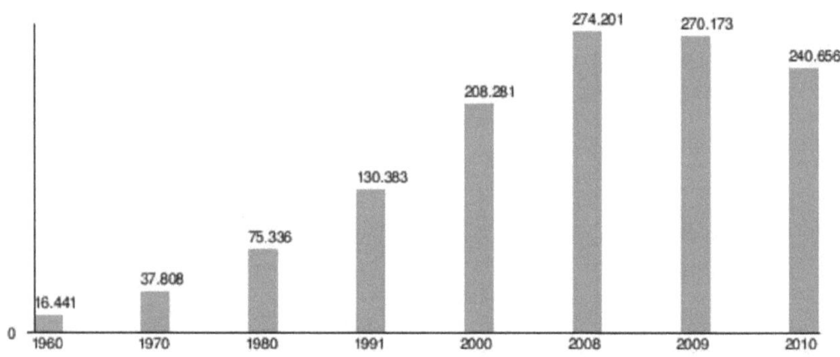

(Source : IBAM)

The Companhia de Saneamento Basico do Estado de Sao Paulo (Sabesp) is responsible for the basic sanitation of the municipality, with a water network extension of 420 km, which covers the entire municipal area, but the sewage network is 270 km long.

Public education in Barueri serves more than 60,000 students, 79 schools and around 2,000 educators (www.barueri.sp.gov.br).

There are 33 secondary schools in the municipality, 23 of which are state public schools, 3 municipal public schools and 7 private schools (IBGE).

Education is considered to be one of the best in the region, and many students from Jandira, Osasco and Carapicuiba go to Barueri to study. The city has 11 libraries, a theater and a museum.

The illiteracy rate of the population aged 15 and over is 6.64% and the *per capita* income of the population is 3.28 minimum wages.

The illiteracy rate is low compared to the rest of the country.

The rate of teenage mothers (under 18) is 7.08% (IBGE).

Barueri's municipal network has 13 basic health units with general dental practitioners.

They work in 4-hour shifts from 7:00 am to 4:00 pm. Only three units have specialists, endodontics and prosthodontics.

The municipality has 36 dental auxiliaries. And there is no oral and maxillofacial emergency care (IBGE, 2005).

The average number of individual basic dental procedures was 0.6 in 2006.

Coverage of the first programmatic dental appointment was 10.4.

The proportion of specialized dental procedures in relation to individual dental actions was 9.3 in 2006 (Datasus, 2006).

The municipality does not yet have epidemiological data on oral health for the adult and elderly populations.

Given the changes in public health policies, which prioritize universal care for all, it is necessary to diagnose the epidemiological profile of all age groups in order to promote health policies that are more egalitarian and non-exclusive.

The Collective Procedures (CP) have been incorporated into the routine of basic health units in the state's municipalities and are mostly applied in elementary schools (1ª to 4ª grade).

It is believed that the permanence of these procedures in schools, together with other factors, contributes to controlling caries rates in children, since the target population becomes part of a prevention system.

The adolescents analyzed reported having had CP at school, but said they didn't know why brushing their teeth prevents caries, gum problems and bad breath.

Expanding PC to adolescents, while they are still at school, could also control the prevalence of oral diseases in this age group.

However, there is resistance on the part of professionals to implementing CP in this age group, especially in its educational component.

There is also resistance from this age group, who don't want to be treated as children or adults.

When evaluating the perception, knowledge, oral health practices and prevalence of caries in adolescents from the municipality of Embu, São Paulo, there was no difference between the groups that did or did not take part in collective procedures as children.

The CPs were not enough to overcome the effects produced by other determinants of the health-disease process and have a favorable impact on future generations (Souza et al., 2007; Junqueira, 2007).

Great emphasis has been placed on evaluating interventions in health services and, consequently, demonstrating their medium and long-term impacts and effects on the population's health levels.

However, according to Watt et al. (2001), there is a gap in the process of evaluating health promotion actions, whether due to a lack of preparation and knowledge in the execution of research in this area by those carrying out the actions, inadequate provision of resources, time and support for evaluation activities or the lack of an appropriate evaluation structure.

The growing concern with research into aspects related to adolescent health is aimed at establishing and maintaining acceptable health conditions, including oral health, as well as helping to demystify certain traditionally accepted assumptions (Flores and Drehmer, 2003; Santos et al., 2007; Gushi et al., 2008; Antunes et al., 2008).

The young people of Barueri believe that when they are adults they will be more careful with their diet and health. They say they are too lazy to take care of themselves, but even so, they brush their teeth two or three times a day, because they are worried about their aesthetics and the demands of their peers.

Prevention systems are defined as "social processes that combine different periodic programmatic actions of a preventive and educational nature in order to control and/or reduce the level of oral diseases affecting a given population or specific social group" (Frazao and Narvai, 1996).

Determining what motivates adolescents is the first step towards successful oral health education (DeBIASE, 1991) and prevention systems.

4.2. Epidemiological survey of Barueri

In Brazil, in 1986, the DMFT at the age of 12 was 6.65, which is a very high prevalence according to the World Health Organization (WHO).

In 1996, an epidemiological oral health survey carried out in all Brazilian capitals showed an average DMFT of 3.06 at the age of 12, which was very close to the target set for the year 2000 by the WHO (DMFT < 3.0).

Currently, approximately 70.0% of the world's countries have reached the target of DMFT < 3.0 by the age of 12 (Word Health Organization, 2006).

The following tables are from the epidemiological survey of oral health conditions in the municipality of Barueri in 2009, carried out by the specialization course in public health at FO-USP.

TABLE 1 - Number of permanent teeth cleaned, decayed, lost and filled, according to age, municipality of Barueri, SP, 2009.

AGE	N	H	C	P	O	CPO
12	3637	3494	83	4	56	143
15-19	2035	1726	127	32	150	309

TABLE 2 - Percentage composition of the DMFT index, according to age, municipality of Barueri, SP. 2009.

AGE	N	C	P	O	CPO
12	133	58.05	2.80	39.16	100,00
15-19	72	41.10	10.36	48.54	100,00

TABLE 3 - Number and percentage of teeth without and with dental treatment needs, according to age, municipality of Barueri, SP, 2009.

AGE	TREATMENT NEEDS				TOTAL	
	SEM		COM			
	n	%	N	%	n	%
5	4560	93,2	331	6,8	4891	100,0
12	3377	96,5	122	3,5	3499	100.0
15-19	1872	92,8	145	7,2	2017	100,0

TABLE 4 - Number and percentage of people examined, according to the highest degree of periodontal condition observed in the individual, by age. Municipality of Barueri, SP, 2009.

CONDITION PERIODONTAL	AGE 12		15 ~ 19		35 ~ 44		65 ~ 74	
	n	%	N	%	n	%	n	%
0 (SADIOS)	37	27,8	13	19,1	24	17,0	10	23,8
1 (BLEEDING)	62	46,6	16	23,5	11	7,8	-	-
2 (CALCULATION)	34	25,6	32	47,1	62	44,0	19	45,2
3 (POCKET 4-5 mm)	-	-	7	10,3	35	24,8	8	19,0
4 (POCKET 6 mm +)	-	-	-	-	9	6,4	5	11,9
X (NULL)	-	-	-	-	-	-	-	-
TOTAL	133	100,0	68	100,0	141	100,0	42	100,0

TABLE 5 - Number and percentage of individuals according to age and degree of fluorosis, municipality of Barueri, SP, 2009.

CONDITION	12		15 ~ 19	
	N	%	n	%
Fluorosis-free	91	68,5	47	65,2
□ Normal	80	60,2	42	58,3
□ Questionable	11	8,3	5	6,9
With Fluorosis	42	31,6	23	32,0
□ Very light	25	18,8	11	15,3
□ Lightweight	11	8,3	11	15,3
□ Moderate	6	4,5	1	1,4
□ Severe	-	-	-	-
No InformationZExcluded			2	2,8
TOTAL	133	100,0	72	100,0

TABLE 6 - Frequency distribution of people examined, by household and age, municipality of Barueri, SP, 2009.

Housing AGE	35 ~ 44	65 ~ 74

	15 ~	19				
	n	%	N	%	n	%
You don't know	-	-	1	0.7	2	2.4
Own	35	48.6	83	56.1	49	58.3
Transferred	8	11.1	21	14.2	16	19.0
Rented	26	36.1	37	25.0	16	19.0
Other	3	4.2	6	4.1	1	1.2
S. inform.	-	-	-	-	-	-
TOTAL	72	100.0	148	100.0	84	100.0

TABLE 7 - Number and percentage of people examined, according to age and number of rooms per dwelling, municipality of Barueri, SP, 2009.

Number of people in the household	15 - 19		35 - 44		65 - 74	
	n	%	N	%	n	%
1-2	11	15.3	18	12.2	41	48.8
3-4	29	40.3	86	58.1	28	33.3
5-10	30	41.7	42	28.4	15	17.9
11 - 15	-	-	1	0.7	-	-
16-20	-	-	-	-	-	-
20 or more	-	-	-	-	-	-
S inform.	2	2.8	1	0.7	-	-
TOTAL	72	100.0	148	100.0	84	100.0

TABLE 8 - Number and percentage of people examined, according to cigarette use and age group, municipality of Barueri, SP, 2009.

Smoking	15 ~ 19		35 ~ 44		65 ~ 74	
	n	%	N	%	n	%
Doesn't smoke and has	64	88,8	94	63,5	25	43,8

never smoked					
Ex-smoker	1	1,38	31	20,9	24	42,1
Smoker - Industrialized Cigarettes	7	9,7	23	15,5	5	8,7
Smoker - Cigarette Straw					2	3,5
Smoker - Pipe					1	1,75
TOTAL	72	100	148	100	57	100

TABLE 9 - Number and percentage of people examined, according to alcohol consumption and age group, municipality of Barueri, SP, 2009.

Frequency of consumption of alcohol	15 ~ 19		35 ~ 44		65 ~ 74	
	n	%	N	%	n	%
Does not ingest and has never	47	65,2	100	67,5	34	59,6
No more eating	3	4,1	17	11,4	8	14
Eat less than once a day	17	23,6	25	16,8	11	19,2
Take 1 to 2 times a day	5	6,9	5	3,3	3	5,2
Eat 3 to 4 times a day			1	0,6	1	1,7
TOTAL	72	100	148	100	57	100

In the epidemiological survey carried out in Barueri in 2009, o CPOD of 15-19 year olds was 4.9 and 7.2 % needed dental treatment.

The periodontal condition drew even more attention as it showed bleeding in 23.5%, calculus in 47.1% and pockets of 4-5mm in 10.3% of the adolescents.

No adolescent had severe fluorosis and 1.4% had moderate fluorosis.

Access to dental services by this age group is divided into 28.6% public, 15.8% private and 37.5% health insurance.

The perception of these young people in relation to their teeth and gums is good for 41.7% and for 87.5% teeth and gums do not affect their relationship. 93.1% report needing dental treatment.

According to Narvai et al. (2000) the factors identified as probably responsible for the decline in the prevalence of caries in Brazil are: the increase and universalization of people's exposure to fluoride in its various forms of application, with special emphasis on the water supply and fluoridated dentifrices, the greater emphasis on health promotion activities, the improvement in health conditions and quality of life, as well as the change in the criteria for diagnosing caries.

This high caries rate among adolescents in Barueri can be explained by the high consumption of sugars and carbohydrates reported by the adolescents, the fragmentation of meals and the lack of care after eating.

Truin et al. (2002) found that although dental caries is the most studied oral disease worldwide, most research focuses on school-age children and there is not enough data in the literature on the prevalence of dental caries in adolescents.

Bratthall et al. (2000) showed a more detailed analysis of the caries situation in many countries.

There is an asymmetrical distribution of caries prevalence - meaning that a proportion of the population still has high DMFT values, while another proportion is completely caries-free.

The average DMFT does not reflect this asymmetrical distribution and could lead to the incorrect conclusion that the caries situation for the entire population is under control, when in reality many individuals still have caries.

Gushi et al.(2002) showed that in the third of the population with the highest rates of dental caries, there was access to dental services, due to the high percentage of restored teeth; However, there was a considerable percentage of missing teeth, demonstrating that often the lack of public services offering quality treatment and the low per *capita* income of the population, which ends up only having lower-cost treatments as an alternative, or the simple lack of access to adequate treatment, can make tooth extraction the only possible course of action.

Consequently, there is a need to emphasize strategies that can mitigate the damage caused by the progression of the disease, such as preventive measures and structured public health programs that meet this demand.

Martins et al. observed in the municipality of Bilac, São Paulo, that the DMFT indices are declining and the percentage of adolescents free of tooth decay is increasing, despite the fact that the municipality does not have fluoridated water supplies.

Baldani et al. found a negative correlation between DMFT and the percentage of households connected to the water supply network in the state of Paranà, indicating lower levels of aggravation in municipalities with a greater supply of water services.

According to Nadanovsky (2000), fluoridated water seems to offer an additional benefit, even when toothpastes contain fluoride.

Sales-Peres and Bastos (2002) in their study in the central-western region of the state of São Paulo, found that there was no significant difference between the DMFT of municipalities of the same size, with or without fluoride in the water, demonstrating the phenomenon of convergence in this region.

This can be explained by the halo effect, which is the exposure of individuals to different fluorine-containing vehicles.

Gushi et al. (2005) found that in municipalities with fluoridation of the public water supply the DMFT index was 6.43 and in municipalities without this benefit the index was 6.45, finding no statistical difference when comparing them ($p = 0.656$).

There was, however, a higher percentage of caries-free adolescents in municipalities with fluoridated water, a trend confirmed by the results obtained from the analysis of the components of the DMFT index, since these municipalities had a lower number of decayed and missing teeth, as well as a higher number of filled teeth.

The decline in cholera rates in several countries has been accompanied by a process of polarization of the disease in a small part of the population.

They remain excluded from the benefits, either because the most important collective health measures (fluoridated water and toothpaste) have not yet reached this segment, or because the conditions of social exclusion and risk of canker have remained at extremely high levels (Antunes, 2006).

4.3. Adolescents' perceptions

The study assessed the needs of these adolescents according to their oral perception.

The opinion of these adolescents, according to certain themes, allowed us to evaluate the context in which they are inserted, their beliefs, customs and expectations for the future.

The analysis of the Barueri adolescents' dialog resulted in the categories that will be discussed below, divided into male and female genders:

Category 1: Adolescents' diets

Category 2: Work

Category 3: Dating

Category 4: Body care

Category 5: Oral hygiene

And these categories will be discussed.

4.3.1.   Category 1: Adolescents' diets

This category discusses adolescents' opinions on food, needs, consumption and the portioning of certain foods.

It was possible to observe that the diet for both groups was high in carbohydrates, sugars, soft drinks and low water consumption.

Mascolino genus:

"The diet has to be balanced." (individual 1)

"To eat well is to be satisfied." (individual 1)

"Eating every 3 minutes is enough." (individual 1)

"[...] If there's nothing to do, I eat." (individual 2)

"[...] Sometimes early, then early again, early again." (individual 2)

"[...] When my hand doesn't leave food ready, I make rice or macaroni, otherwise I make Miojo, make a farofa with meat and eat it." (individual 3)

"[...] Maçâ can only eat when he's at home, because people who wear braces are bad, their braces get dirty." (individual 4)

"[...] At home, my father comes home with different fruit all the time [...] I've never eaten it." (individual 4)

"I eat all day if I let myself." (individual 5)

"[...] If there's food, I eat it, then I nibble on cheese, mortadella, ham, straight Pâo.

I eat sweets [...] every day when I get home from school." (individual 5)

Female gender

"At home it's a lot of salad, a lot of vegetables, a lot of healthy things." (individual 1)

"Ah, at home we never worried about food, these things, so much so that my mother has hemorrhage, I also have a kidney stone, when we see it, ah, we want it, we eat it. There's never been any of that. I hate salad, I've never eaten salad, I hate salad, there's nothing vegetable about it and stuff. And there's no time to eat either." (individual 2)

"In my house you have to eat lunch and dinner every day. My father is like that, if my mother doesn't cook she's already lazy, so we have to eat all our meals properly. But we also eat a lot of junk food. My father is a lifelong chocoholic, cookies, soft drinks, chewing gum, candy, lots of it." (individual 3)

"I'm already thin, there's no such thing. When I eat I eat a lot, but also when I don't want to eat I don't eat. Today I haven't eaten anything all day and I'm not hungry at all." (Individual 4)

"There's a lot of junk food at home too. I try to look after my body, so sometimes I don't eat dinner because I know it's fattening. I train in martial arts, so I don't eat because I lose weight in training, I lose my hunger in training." (Individual 5)

"[...] I like chocolate a lot, sweets, here at school it's candy all day long." (Individual 6)

"[...] At home the only meal that is certain is lunch, dinner is if you feel like eating. There's no day to order snacks, pizza, yesterday it was pizza, we order Friday. Lunch isn't lunch at home if there's no Coke. Nobody drinks coffee. And I live on chocolate." (Individual 7)

"[...] My parents don't like eating junk food, but I do. At weekends, they sometimes eat pizza and snacks. We don't have much time to eat either, we eat when we feel like it. And I love eating sweets." (Individual 8)

"At home, on weekdays, I don't eat lunch, I only eat dinner. I like to eat candy, sweets, candy practically all day. I also like to eat chocolate [...]" (individual 9)

"But it's because when you're a teenager, it's all about junk food, potato chips, cola, chocolate, you take the money and go straight out and buy what? Chocolate. You're sad, what are you going to eat? ChocolateC (individual 4)

Adolescence is considered a vulnerable phase in nutritional terms, mainly because there is a greater demand for nutrients, related to the dramatic increase in physical growth and development, lifestyle changes and inadequate eating habits, affecting nutrient intake and needs.

In addition, participation in sports, pregnancy, the development of eating disorders, excessive dieting, the use of alcohol and drugs are common situations in adolescents' lives and can further compromise their nutritional status (Mahan and Scott-Stump, 2002).

According to Fisberg et al. (2000), the main problems detected in adolescents' diets are:

■ Omission of meals, especially breakfast, which can lead to lower school performance;

Replacing the main meals (lunch and dinner) with snacks, especially when this is the family habit;

■ High intake of soft drinks (approximately one liter per day);

■ Foods with a high calorie density (usually fried snacks, filled cookies, chocolate and a high consumption of sweets on a daily basis);

Low intake of fruit and vegetables.

It is known that during the period of peak growth velocity, adolescents often need to consume larger quantities of food, being able to use them with a high concentration of energy.

However, they need to be more careful with the frequency of feeding once growth has ceased.

Binge eating habits adopted during adolescence can ultimately contribute to a series of debilitating diseases, as well as overweight and obesity (Mahan and Scott-Stump, 2002).

4.3.2. Category 2: Work: expectations for the future

From the speeches it was possible to see that work for boys is much more common.

The majority had already worked and were more certain about what they wanted for their professional future, while the girls knew they wanted to study, but were uncertain about what to do and the majority had never worked.

Male gender

"Work, only in 2012 for me. Next year I'll go to ITB, then 2^0 year of ITB they'll give you an internship. So, for me, it's not until 2012." (Individual 4)

"I worked as a bricklayer, a bricklayer's assistant." (individual 2)

"I have a rock band, so I earn a few bucks when we perform." (individual 6)

"I clean the house, I do general cleaning. My mother doesn't give me any money, but if I ask her for something, she gives it to me." (individual 4)

"[...] I've worked in a tire shop, as a bricklayer's assistant." (individual 7)

"I don't know yet." (Individual 3)

"I have two plans. To pursue a career as a civil engineer or in IT." (Individual 5)

"I'm going into computer science and robotics." (individual 1) "In engineering or electronics." (Individual 8)

Female gender

"I'm not thinking about a job now. I've never worked. I'm going to start a technical course next year. I still don't know what I'm going to do with my life, I'm still thinking." (Individual 9)

"I've never worked. I don't know what I'm going to do, I'm still thinking. I'm going to do normal high school, but I don't know yet." (Individual 10)

"I'm also going to do a technical course, but at the moment I'm just thinking about studying, I've never worked either. Over time, you get traineeships, you learn and so on. I'm going to study administration." (Individual 8)

"I'm going to do technical training next year, but I don't know what I want to do yet. I change my mind very easily, so I don't even think about it because the more I think about it, the more I change my mind, so I'm keeping it quiet and when I go to work I'll look into it, but for now I haven't thought about it. I've never worked. I'm going to become a building technician." (Individual 7)

"I've never worked. I'm also going to study building technology, and for my future I want to take the USP exam and get into medicine." (Individual 6)

"I'm going to do a technical course too, administration. If I had to choose what I really wanted, it would be to be a footballer. That's what I wanted most. I could also be a businesswoman, so I'm going to study a lot. I've never worked, I've only been a teacher, teaching a boy there, cleaning my grandmother's house." (Individual 5)

"[...] I'm also going to do buildings, because it involves mathematics and I love mathematics, I love problems, equations, roots, all that stuff that everyone runs away from, I love it. And I don't know if I'm going to go into buildings, I think I'm going to be an engineer or something, if I don't die by then (laughs). I've worked looking after babies, but it's my sister, so I didn't get paid, so for me it's not a job. You work, you work hard, but you get nothing, so it's worth nothing." (individual 4)

"I kind of work, I make websites. I've already done a web design course, I'm going to continue, I'm going to do computer science on the internet, a technical course as well. I want to be a photographer, my father already wanted to open a studio for me, but no, calm down, in three years we'll open a studio for me. I want to go to university too, I've already done a web design course, I've finished it, I'm doing another one on making flyers, these things, I already know how to do them too." (Individual 2)

"I don't work, I'm going to study administration. I'm thinking of working in this area, but right now I'm just studying, I have no certain future." (individual 1)

"I've never worked. I'm going to study computer science and I intend to go on, but I really want to do business administration. I've never worked outside. " (Individual 11)

"I've never worked, I'm going to ITB next year, I'm going to do a computer science degree online. And I only think about studying, I don't have anything prepared like that. I wanted to be a teacher, but I've changed my mind." (Individual 8)

According to data from the 2000 census, there are around 9 million teenagers aged between 15 and 19 who are in the labor market (IBGE).

For teenagers, work has a deeper meaning, closely linked to maturity and economic emancipation.

Early work generally has negative effects on physical and educational development, preventing young people from engaging in extracurricular activities such as leisure and social activities appropriate to their age, isolating young people from their peers and families, and causing them to fall behind at school.

Becker (1987) explains that adolescence can be better understood as a passage that produces a change of attitude in the individual who, from being a mere spectator, assumes a more active and questioning stance towards life.

It is a period of review, self-criticism and transformation and a vital phase in a person's development process.

In this sense, it can be seen as a process during which, slowly and gradually, the subject matures in an attempt to achieve individuation and build their own identity (Coleman, 1979; Pais, 2003).

Access to employment is becoming especially difficult for teenagers as a result of structural unemployment.

Alongside the increase in the number of teenagers and young people in the population as a whole, they are more unstable in their jobs and stay there less than their older colleagues.

High turnover limits the accumulation of professional experience, which makes it difficult to find a new job (Seade, 1998).

Data obtained in the Sao Paulo Metropolitan Region in 1996 indicates that previous work experience and a higher level of schooling contribute to the entry of 15 to 24 year olds into the productive system, to their remaining in employment, and to better pay and shorter working hours.

Despite this, schooling alone does not guarantee a job, given that 23% of the inactive or unemployed had completed secondary school.

Schooling can also lead to the expectation of a job, which, however, is not always realized (Seade, 1998).

Even so, data from the 2000 IBGE Demographic Census shows a directly proportional relationship between the number of years of schooling and income (IBGE, 2004).

4.3.3. Category 3: Love relationships in the adoleseene

In these speeches, it was possible to observe that these adolescents are healthy, happy and willing to have an emotional relationship, whether it is a fixed relationship or not.

Mascolino genus:

"I had a fight with my girlfriend on Friday." (individual 6)

"You know everything about the girl, her faults - I don't know - you can't." (Individual 5)

"It's harassment, it doesn't work. These girls are worse than us. We rarely go to them to ask them to stay with us. It's usually them. At least I'm like that, I don't run after them. [...] Also, dating is a waste of time, start dating now. Staying with someone for a while, a couple of weeks, that's fine, but staying for two years, three years, that's not good. One, because I don't have any money. I can't afford a girl." (Individual 4)

"As soon as I entered the school, a girl asked me to stay, I stayed, then there was a fuss, the principal found out, I was almost expelled." (Individual 7)

"I've been with a girl from school, but hidden. If the principal finds out... (laughs) In the classroom." (Individual 4)

"The Portuguese teacher is a bit mad about ideas. She doesn't see. We go out in her class, do what we want and she doesn't even see it. She doesn't pay attention." (Individual 6)

Female gender:

"I think all men are no good[...] I've already dated for 1 year and 4 months, I'm 15, so I started dating when I was 12[...] If women are complicated, men are twice as complicated. That's all. I'm still a virgin, I'm not ashamed to say it." (Individual 4)

"I'm dating, on the 4th it's been 1 year and 8 months. It's really complicated, too much. My father still doesn't accept it. He doesn't even want to see him painted gold, he saw him once and thought he was ridiculous. Dad's crazy.[...] I started dating early, but it wasn't my first. It's the first one that works out, that goes ahead, but the others weren't boyfriends, it was kissing there, kissing, but I was never much of a fan, if I were to put it on my fingers, there were only five boys. Every year I fall in love with one. So this time it worked out and it's going." (individual 2)

"I'm not dating. I broke up a while ago because it didn't work out. I've had four boyfriends and none of them worked out. Men are no good to me either. I don't want to. My thing is to stay put." (Individual 4)

"I've been dating for 2 years and 1 month, at home, serious, cute, my mom and dad know. Now, my father let me, it was also like the case of individual 2, he wouldn't let me, he knew, but he wouldn't accept any waste, but now, about 3 months ago, he let me, he talked to him, everything.

" (individual 1)

"I've never dated and I'm not thinking about it. No, I don't. I want to study first, then think about men." (individual 11)

"Oh, I suck. I like a boy, we've been going out, then he asks me out, then I say yes, then some people come up to me and say, 'Oh, he's such a prick, if I were you I'd break up, you're such a prick'". (Individual 6)

"I used to date seriously, but now I'm taking a break. I started early, but... I was with a guy for a while, about two years, going back and forth, trying, it didn't work out, trying, it didn't work out. My father and mother think I've never kissed. If my father finds out, he'll kill me. I'd better keep to myself." (Individual 7)

"I'd have the courage to go to the gynecologist, but my mother doesn't talk to me about it, so..." (individual 4)

"My mother didn't, as soon as I started dating [...] she took me to the gynecologist. The gynecologist said to me: if all mothers were like yours, many children would have been avoided. And my mother said, I don't have to believe that you won't do it, because I know you will, so (laughs) And I take contraceptives." (individual 1)

The concepts of puberty and adolescence are not synonymous. Puberty is a set of physical transformations, of growth and maturation of the body, which transform boys and girls into people with reproductive capacity; it is a universal phenomenon that must occur in all individuals, regardless of culture, social class, educational level or other psychosocial differences.

It is with Puberty that the period of Adolescence begins, characterized as a period that involves a set of social roles with psychological repercussions directly related to the social group to which the subject belongs and the historical moment in which they live; therefore, adolescence is a cultural phenomenon (Maia, 2003).

Puberty is marked by an increase in the production of sex hormones.

With hormonal influence, the bodies of boys and girls begin to show changes, both in the growth of organs and in the maturation of their functions.

The pattern of growth and maturation, following functional changes in the hypothalamic-pituitary axis, depends mainly on changes in the functioning of the endocrine gland system, influenced by various environmental factors that have a direct impact on the individual's general state of health (Goodson and Diaz, 1990).

In girls, the essential hormones are estrogen and progesterone, and the characteristics developed are: a) breast enlargement, b) the appearance of pubic and axillary hair, c) the occurrence of menarche, d) greater sexual eroticization through vaginal lubrication and, finally e) the ability to reproduce.

In boys, the essential hormone is testosterone and the characteristics are: a) the growth of the testicle, b) the appearance of pubic and axillary hair, c) the enlargement of the penis, d) a change in the voice, e) ejaculations, first without and later with the production of spermatozoa, f) the appearance of a beard, g) an increase in sexual drive, aggressiveness and physical strength, h) growth in stature and, finally i) the beginning of the ability to reproduce.

For teenagers, dating can be a source of pleasure as well as anxiety and conflict.

Generally, a lack of experience in romantic relationships leads to anguish and inappropriate fantasies.

The boy is socially expected to take the initiative and be able to "teach" the girl, when in fact he is also unaware of various aspects of the affective and sexual relationship (Rodrigues, 1993).

Abandoning the "security" of a group of friends in order to enter into a romantic relationship is not an easy task for either sex, generating anxiety, as it is necessary to abandon a stable relationship in the "clique" in order to develop a new role as a lover (Monesi, 1993).

4.3.4.   Category 4: Body care

It can be seen in the discourse that caring for one's body appears to be a demonstration of good health. The vast majority of adolescents, regardless of gender, reported doing some kind of exercise.

Body care is limited to bathing and sports.

Male gender:

"I take care of my body a lot[...]I shower, brush my teeth, I get a lot of pimples, but I use a cream." (individual 7)

"I play float. I play volleyball. I play video games. That's it. And I sleep. I wake up, shower and go to school." (Individual 9)

"Oh, I shower. Every time I go out I do a workout, something like that. I cut my hair. I use a little machine, sometimes my stepfather. I take a shower, put on some cream and go out, normal. When I get back, I shower." (individual 2)

"Sport, I do soccer and swimming." (Individual 8)

"Nowadays, it doesn't pay to study, it pays to play ball from an early age. If you learn to play ball, you'll earn 5OO thousand a month." (Individual 4)

"When I come to school I take a shower, when I leave school I take another one. I stay at home, when my mother comes with my brother-in-law we go out, we go fishing. [...]" (individual 3)

"When I go off to school I have a shower, when I come back from school I have another shower, then sometimes the kids in the street call me to play ball in the street, I take a cap off my finger (laughs), I shave it all off, I ride my bike. That's it." (individual 1)

"I wake up, brush my teeth, go to buy bread, take a shower to go to school, when I get there, I take another shower, I stay out until about 9:30, when I come back, I take another shower. And I used to do volleyball, but I don't anymore because I was on the court, here, playing, the boy came and stepped on my foot, broke my foot, now I'm doing therapy on my tendon" (individual 3).

"Also. I play soccer, volleyball, everything, any sport that calls me, I go. If it calls me, I do it. What I don't like is sitting still. Body care, I shower too much, if you look at it, I shower five or six times a day. It's very hot, I get dirty very easily. Two brothers have to stay on the street, we get carried away and go with them. These days I arrived, it was raining, me and my classmates were in the mud, the 15-, 16-year-olds playing in the mud. In the old days, I was fresher, I used to put foundation on my nails, nowadays, I don't even have nails anymore, I used to put cream on them." (Individual 6)

Female gender:

"I walk around a bit. Sometimes I go to the bus stop and back. (laughs) Sometimes I play ball, sometimes volleyball, sometimes I play with my dog. On Saturdays I swim. That's it" (individual 1)

"I walk a lot, sometimes I walk from Carapicuiba. It's a long way, an hour to walk. Although I go by car. Then on Saturdays and Sundays I don't leave the house because I walk, I stay at home, with all the walking I do, I get tired. That's all I'm saying. Sometimes I go to the park with my brothers, to walk with them. They don't leave the house, they just go to school and come back, my mother doesn't like going out much, so I take them to the park near my house. (individual 11)

"I like dancing a lot too, I dance. I love playing sports, I love soccer, I love volleyball, I love handball, I'm always playing something, the ball is... I love playing ball. I've also done swimming. I run a lot, but because I have a kidney stone I get tired very quickly and start to feel pain, so I can't run much, or play sports, but I love it. Whenever I can I play, I swim." (Individual 2)

"Look, I'm the one who talks about doing sport. I play a bit of everything, I play with the boys, soccer on the court, I run to one side, I come out all red-faced, just don't throw me in the pool or I'll drown. I don't know anything, I don't think I can float either. I used to do volleyball, but that ended this week, twice a week, then all of Physical Education I play soccer with the boys, I run to one side and the other, I look like a fool chasing the ball. Basketball isn't my thing. I play volleyball, handball and the school championship. I don't know anything about swimming, I'd drown."

(Individual 4)

"I play soccer. I don't like volleyball or basketball, just soccer and handball. I fight kung fu. Then, when I think my body is getting out of shape, I start eating salad." (Individual 5)

"I like to play soccer, a lot, at the weekend, every day, in the street playing. I've done swimming. I've done judo. I've played soccer on the pitch. I like cycling, I like doing everything, playing everything, except volleyball and basketball, because I'm short, that doesn't work. I shower every day." (Individual 9)

When a healthy child is between 9 and 16 years old, he or she enters puberty.

The exact age depends on factors such as heredity, nutrition and whether the child is a boy or a girl.

On average, boys enter puberty 2 years later than girls.

At this point, the pituitary and hypothalamus glands (endocrine glands) start sending out new hormones that trigger the changes of puberty.

General changes in boys and girls include sudden increases in height and weight, the development of secondary sexual characteristics (the appearance of an adult woman or man) and increased sexual interest (sex drive).

In girls, the ovaries begin to increase their production of estrogen and other "female" hormones. In boys, the testicles increase their production of testosterone.

The sweat glands become more active and the sweat produced has a slightly different content than when the child was small (more than one odor begins to appear).

The oil glands become more active and acne can appear.

At this point, the importance of personal hygiene becomes apparent and it is important for boys and girls who are becoming mature to pay attention to regular bathing and other aspects of hygiene.

The loss of virginity is still an important milestone for young people.

It is a rite of sexual initiation, which can be experienced with pride or excessive guilt, depending on the family's upbringing and tradition.

Initially, young people only seek sexual involvement, testing their new abilities and reactions to previously unknown sensations.

It's the rediscovery of the body. Only afterwards do they seek complementary emotional involvement, starting to live together not only in packs, but also in pairs.

In adolescence, the construction of personal identity necessarily includes the relationship with one's own body; and this relationship is made through the mental representation that young people have of their bodies, in other words, through their body image (Ferriani et al., 2005).

4.3.5.   Category 5: Oral hygiene

In the discourse, we observed that oral hygiene for adolescents is the number of times they brush their teeth (2 to 3 times a day) and whether they go to a private dentist or one with a health insurance.

Male gender:

"When I was in grade 4[a] I broke my tooth twice, this tooth here (shows a front tooth). It broke. Once, I was walking backwards and a kid knocked me down, I fell on my mouth. Another time, I was in the bathroom at school, there was a kid in the bathroom, I locked the door and ran out, the kid jumped over the door, ran out and hit me, I fell and broke the same tooth, again[...]The bad thing about braces is brushing, with braces you can't brush your teeth properly. You can't. You have to spend half an hour brushing your teeth. The most important brushing I do is at bedtime, [...]" (individual 5)

"I brush my teeth when I wake up, after I've had my coffee, when I go to school and when I go to sleep." (Individual 8)

"When I was 7 years old I was playing hopscotch, then a girl, she didn't mean to, she grabbed me and pushed me, and I broke five of my front teeth. It took a while to grow in, it only grew in after the age of 8. Then, when I was 12, I went to the dentist and he said I had to have my teeth cleaned, because when I was little I ate a lot of toothpaste, so I had to have my teeth cleaned when I was 15. Now, it wouldn't work because it's too crazy." (individual 3)

"I broke a tooth when I was 8 years old. I broke this one (shows a front tooth). I broke it with the flute, I was playing the flute, then the dog came and hit my leg, my leg was soft, I hit it, the flute hit the wall and hit my mouth. Then the tooth didn't get soft, it usually gets soft, mine didn't get soft, it just broke the tooth and bled around the tooth" (individual 5).

"There was one time when I was holding a vacuum cleaner pipe like this (showing my arms) and pushing it on the floor with my mouth, then there was a little gap in the floor, the thing got tangled up and I went forward, hit my gum, a ball came out and my gum turned black, I just don't remember if I went to the private dentist or the public one. Then he pulled it out, my milk tooth fell out, it fell out, there was a black ball here, it got inflamed. I don't remember if I went to a private or public dentist.[...] I'm afraid of injections, the ones they stick in your mouth." (Individual 4)

"I started punching them. They didn't want to leave, so I got angry and punched them, almost swallowing them." (individual 1)

"Oh, I can't remember the last time I went to the dentist. It's been a while. I think I need to see if everything is all right" (individual 7).

"You feel that, men at least, I don't know girls, men worry about their mouths for only one reason: girls. That's the only reason. I don't know, girl." (Individual 4)

"My aunt said that while you're eating you have to brush." (individual 1)

"Yes. I'm the one who takes the most care of the family. On my father's side, not many. My cousin wakes up and goes straight to the computer. The other goes straight to the carpet. The aunts, straight to baking. The uncles, straight to work. I'm the only one who takes good care. My father, his teeth are like this (shows with his hands), they look like a V, my mother's teeth are yellow like this curtain there, but a little more turns them blue" (individual 2).

"In the past there was a lack of information. There wasn't as much information as there is today. Mothers didn't tell their children to brush their teeth like they do today." (Individual 4)

Female

"I don't have a toothache. I haven't been to the dentist for ages." (Individual 9)

"I don't know. (laughs) I've never been to the dentist. I've never felt pain, nothing." (individual 2)

"I've never been to the dentist either, I've never had a toothache. I brush my teeth three times a day, I can't sleep without brushing my teeth or have breakfast. I consider my hygiene to be good. I also shower before going to school and afterwards. That's it." (individual 5)

"I brush my teeth only before I go to school and to bed, I don't brush my teeth in the morning, I'm too lazy, I don't floss, I'm too lazy. I shower, of course. I can't go a day without showering. I go to the dentist from time to time, but I've been a lot, I've had cavities, I've broken my tooth, it's still broken today, I don't go. That's it." (individual 3) "I brush my teeth 2 or 3 times a day. I shower twice, on my way to and from school. I haven't been to the dentist for a long time, but I don't have any problems with my teeth, no pain, I'm not afraid of the dentist." (individual 11)

"I still think we have a conscience, it's just laziness." (individual 3)

"I'm in love with a beautiful smile. I think it's beautiful. For me, a smile is a calling card." (individual 1)

"Because my parents smoke, I want to stay away. My father doesn't have any teeth in his mouth, he has two to hold his dentures, that's all. My mother is all yellow, she wears braces, now she's taken them off, they're back on, everything's crooked again, and I don't want that. They both smoke. She's stopped now because of my brother, but..." (individual 7)

"At a party, the main thing is booze. For our age, a party without booze isn't a party." (Individual 4)

"I've drunk champagne, I really like champagne, but only my father and mother don't know. I mean, my dad doesn't know that I've had it, that I've tried it because he gave it to me. (laughs)" (individual 10)

"A party at home at the end of the year, my father offers it to me, he says: I'd rather you start drinking at home than start on the street and get hooked at once, stay at home, drink a little bit [...]" (individual 7)

"There's a lot of booze at home, a lot. There's a cupboard full of wine, there's another cupboard full of glasses, glasses of everything, glasses of wine, glasses of whisky, glasses of pinga, glasses of everything, there's a lot of drink. It's just that my father, he offers it to me every time he has a drink: do you want it? No, thank you. I don't drink with him, only once in a while, at parties and so on. But he drinks a lot. My mother tries to follow him from time to time, but she ends up falling asleep, dying of sleep, she can't do it, she can't take it like him." (individual 1)

Sheiham (2004) argues that most young people clean their teeth regularly because brushing is associated with good looks.

Dental hygiene is also related to young people's concern with personal hygiene, the feeling of freshness and good breath (Lisboa and Abegg, 2006).

We can't forget the existing advertisements, especially in magazines, which indirectly claim that physical appearance is responsible for happiness and success (Thomsen et al., 2002).

Cultural values related to aesthetics and greater access to health information are more evident in social classes with higher purchasing power, which may justify the fact that adolescents from private schools cite teeth and hair as very important (Campos et al., 2003; Granville-Garcia et al., 2008).

The desire to look good is not just a sign of vanity at this stage.

In services considered prestigious, or where there is direct contact with the public, employees must have good dental aesthetics (Jenny and Proshek, 1986).

In a study carried out by Elias et al. (2001), adolescents were concerned about good oral health in order to find jobs. It is extremely important to understand adolescents and their needs, especially so that health or education professionals can make an effort to positively influence this part of the population, who can act as health multipliers.

5. Conclusion

The adolescents were separated into male and female genders, so we were able to notice some of the peculiar behaviors of each sex.

The girls go into much more detail on each subject, always answering and asking questions in greater depth.

Boys, on the other hand, want to demonstrate masculinity, virility, are a little more evasive, always have the upper hand and show a very strong link between their actions and the girls they want.

The speeches showed that sexuality and its orientation are subjects that are little discussed among families and in the school.

Discussing the issue of sexuality as something educational, dialoguing between different professionals on how to work with sexuality in different situations would be a great achievement.

I believe that educational proposals on sexuality could make a major contribution to emancipatory sexual education in adolescence and, above all, to promoting a healthy and responsible sex life throughout life.

The study found an increase in the number of cavities in this age group, due to the high intake of carbohydrates.

Oral health for these young people is mainly related to habit.

I believe that educational work aimed specifically at this target group could lead to more efficient results in terms of controlling and reducing tooth decay rates.

There was little demand for public dental services, either due to the spread of health insurance, the belief that public services are mutilating or the lack of need, according to their perceptions.

Cigarettes and alcohol were discussed as risk factors for oral diseases.

But what was striking was how much drinking seemed to be facilitated and not reprimanded by family members.

The frequency of this consumption is reported to be fundamental at their parties and meetings.

As for cigarettes, some said they had tried them but all said they didn't like them.

I believe that raising awareness among young people alone wouldn't be enough, given that stimulation and access are often provided at home.

Changing behavior and understanding the risk that drinking can bring must be incorporated into the daily life of the population as a whole, as it is a cultural problem.

The population is now able to understand the risks posed by cigarettes, but drinking is so widespread and common that the work of raising awareness must be more incisive and permanent.

Knowledge of young people's perceptions of these axes can help to improve oral health actions, which take into account the social determinants of health and how to articulate access to means of prevention, treatment and maintenance of oral health with objective needs (epidemiology) and subjective needs (their own needs).

6. Bibliographical references

1 - Andersen R, Newman JF. Societal and individual determinants of medical care utilization in the United States. MilbankMem Fund Quar 1973; 51:95-124.

2 - Antunes JLF, Peres MA, Frias AC, Crosato EM, Biazevic MGH. Gingival health of adolescents and the use of dental services, State of São Paulo. Revista Saùde Pùblica. Rio de Janeiro,v.42,n.2,p.191-199,2008.

3 - Atchinson KA, Dolan TA. Development of the Geriatric Oral Health Assessment Index. J Dent Educ 1990, 54(11):680-687.

4 - Baldani MH, Narvai PC, Antunes JLF. Dental caries and socioeconomic conditions in the state of Parana, Brazil, 1996. Cad Saùde Pùblica 2002;18(3):755-763.

5 - Bardin L. Content analysis. Lisbon: Ediçoes 70, 1977. 236p.

6 - Berger P I, Luckmann T A. Social construction of reality. Petrópolis: Vozes, 1987. 248 p.

7 - Biazevic MGH, Araùjo ME, Crosato EM. Quality of life indicators related to oral health: a systematic review. UFES Rev Odontol 2002, 4(2):13-25.

8 - Botazzo C . Oral health in the context of the Family Health Strategy: helping to promote health for individuals, groups and families. In: Moysés ST, Kriger L, Moysés SJ. Family oral health: working with evidence. Sâo Paulo: Artes Médicas, 2008. p.81-88.

9 - Brazil. Ministry of Health. Guidelines for the National Oral Health Policy.

Available at URL: http://www.saude.gov.br. Accessed on February 20, 2010.

10 - Brazil. Ministry of Health. National Health Care Secretariat. ABC do SUS - Doctrinas e Principios. Brasilia, 1990.

11 - Brazil. Ministry of Health. Constitution of the Federative Republic of Brazil, 1988.

12 - Brathall D. Introducing the Significant Caries Index Together with a proposal for a new global oral health goal for 12-year-olds.Int.Dent J 2000, 50: 378-84.

13 - Campos JADB , Guimaraes MS . Health education in adolescence.Ciência Odontologica Brasileira.v.6, n.4,p.48-53,2003.

14 - Cardoso L, Rosing C, Kramer P, Costa CC, Costa Filho LC. Caries polarization in a municipality without fluoridated water. Cad Saùde Pùblica 2003;19(1):237-243.

15 - DeBiase CB. Dental health education: theory and practice. Pennsylvania: Lea 7 Febiger, 1991. 314p.

16 - Elias ,MS , Cano MAT , Mastriner Junior, W , Ferriani BGC. The importance of oral health for adolescents from different social strata in Ribeirao Preto. Revista Latino-Americana de Enfermagem.v.9,n.1,p.88-95,2001.

17 - Ferriani MGC , Dias TS , Silvia KZ ,Martins CS .Body self-image of adolescents assisted in a multidisciplinary program of assistance to obese adolescents.Revista Brasileira de saùde materno infantil.v.5,n 1,2005.

18 - Flores EMTL, Drehmer TM. Knowledge, perceptions, behaviors and representations of oral health and disease among adolescents from public schools in two districts of Porto Alegre. Rev C S Col 2003; 8(3):743-752.

19 - Frazao P, Narvai PC. Promoting oral health in schools. Text prepared for course HSP-281/Preventive Dentistry and Public Health given to students of the Dentistry Course at the University of Sao Paulo, 1996.

20 - Godoy, A. S. Pesquisa qualitativa: tipos fundamentais.Revista de Administraçao de Empresas, Sao Paulo, v. 35, n. 3, p. 20-29, maio/jun. 1995.

21 - Granville-Garcia AF, Loreana Sobrinho JE , Menezes VA, Cavalcanti AL . Occurrence of smoking and associated factors in schoolchildren.RFO.v.13,n.1,p.30-34,2008.

22 - Gushi LL ,Soares MC ,Forni TIB ,Vieira V, WadaRS ,Sousa MLR .Dental caries in adolescents aged 15 to 19 in the state of Sao Paulo,2002. Cad. Saùde Pùbçica vol.21 no.5 2005.

23 - Gushi LL, Soares MC, Rihis LB, Forni TIB, Vieira V, Wada RS, Souza MLR. Dental caries and treatment needs in adolescents in the state of Sao Paulo, 1998 and 2002.Revista de Saùde Pùblica.Sao Paulo,v.42,n.3,p.480-486,2008.

24 - Jenny J , Proshek JM .Visibility and prestige of occupations and the importance of dental appearance. Journal of Canadian Dental Association.v.52, n.12,p.987-989,1986.

25 - Junqueira SR. Effectiveness of collective oral health procedures: dental caries in adolescents in Embu, SP, 2005. [Doctoral thesis]. Sao Paulo: USP School of Public Health; 2007.

26 - Laville C, Dionne J. The construction of knowledge. Belo Horizonte: UFMG, 1999. 340 p.

27 - Lisboa IC, Abegg C.Habitos de higiene bucal e uso de serviços odontológicos por adolescentes e adultos do Municipio de Canoas,Estado do Rio Grande do Sul,Brasil. Epidemiologia e Serviços de Saùde.v.15,n.4,p.29-39,2006.

28 - Martins RJ, Garbin CAS, Garbin AJI, Moimaz SAS, Saliba O. Decline of caries in a municipality in the northwest region of the State of Sao Paulo, Brazil, from 1998 to 2004. Cad Saùde Pùblica 2006;22(5):1035-1041

29 - Minayo MCS. The challenge of knowledge: qualitative research in health. Sao Paulo/Rio de Janeiro: Hucitec-ABRASCO, 1998.

30 - Nadanovsky P. The decline of caries. In: Pinto VG, organizer. Collective oral health. Sao Paulo: Santos; 2000. p.341-351

31 - Narvai PC, Castellanos RA, Frazao P. Prevalence of caries in permanent teeth of schoolchildren in the Municipality of Sao Paulo, SP, 1970 - 1996. Rev Saùde Pùblica 2000; 34: 196-200.

32 - Sales-Peres SHC, Bastos JRM. Epidemiological profile of dental caries in 12-year-old children living in fluoridated and non-fluoridated cities in the Midwest region of the State of São Paulo.

Sao Paulo, Brazil. Cad Saùde Pdblica 2002;18(5):1281-1288.

33 - Santos VA, Alves CRA , Ciamponi AL, Corrêa MSNP. Oral health habits in children and adolescents living in the city of Sao Paulo. Rev Odontopediatria v.1, n.3, p.183-193, 1992.

34 - Santos NCN, Alves TDB , Freitas VS, Jamelli SR, Sarinho ESC. The oral health of adolescents: aspects of hygiene, dental caries and periodontal disease in the cities of Recife, Pernambuco and Feira de Santana, Bahia.Ciência & Sadde Coletiva.Rio de Janeiro,v.12,n.5,p.1155-1166,2007.

35 - Sheiham A. Public Health approaches to promoting periodontal health. In: Bonecker M, Sheiham A. Promoting oral health in children and adolescents: knowledge and practice. Sao Paulo: Santos; 2004.

36 - Souza GB, Sa PHRN, Junqueira S, Frias AC. Evaluation of collective oral health procedures: perception of adolescents from Embu, SP. Sadde Soc 2007; 16(3):138-148.

37 - Thomsen SR , Mccoy JK, Gustafson RL, Williams M. Motivations for reading beauty and fashion magazines and anorexic risk in college-age women. Media Psychology.v.2,n.4,p.113-135,2002.

38 - Tomita NE, Pernambuco RA, Lauris JRP, Sampayo E . Oral health education for adolescents: use of participatory methods. Rev Fac Odontol Bauru v.9, n.1, p.63-69, 2001.

39 - Trivinos ANS . Introduction to research in the social sciences: qualitative research in education. Sao Paulo: Atlas, 1987. 175 p.

40 - Watt RG, Fuller S, Harnett R, Treasure ET, Stilman-Lowe C. Oral health promotion evaluation - time for development. Community Dent Oral Epidemiol 2001; 29: 161-166.

41 - World Health Organization. Dental caries levels at 12 years. Geneva: WHO; 1994.

42 - WHO (World Health Organization), 1995. Physical Status: The Use and Interpretation of Anthropometry. WHO Technical Report Series 854. Geneva: WHO.

43 - Barueri (Data from the Municipality of Barueri)(2010).Accessed from www.barueri.sp.gov.br on October 20, 2010.

44 - Datasus (Unified Health System Database) (2010). Accessed from www.datasus.gov.br on October 22, 2010.

45 - IBGE (Brazilian Institute of Geography and Statistics) (2010). Accessed from www.ibge.gov.br on October 22, 2010.

46 - Sabesp (Saneamento Basico do Estado de Sao Paulo) (2010). Accessed from www.sabesp.com.br on October 15, 2010.

47 - Seade (Fundaçao Sistema Estadual de Analise de Dados) (2010). Accessed from www.seade.gov.br on October 15, 2010.

48 - Mahan LK, Escott-Stump S. Alimentos,Nutriçâo eDietoterapia.10^a ed., Sao Paulo: Roca, 2002.

49 - Fisberg M, et al. Eating habits in adolescence. Pediatria Moderna 2000; 36 (11): 724734.

50 - Becker D. O que é adolescència. Sao Paulo: Brasiliense , 1987.

51 - Coleman, J C. Current views of the adolescent process. In: Coleman JC. (Org.) The school years. Current issues in the socialization of young people. London: Methuen , 1979.

52 - Pais J M. Culturas Juvenis. Lisbon: National Press - Casa da Moeda, 2003.

53 - Maia ACB . Sexuality and Disabilities in the School Context. Doctoral thesis. Universidade Estadual Paulista: Marilia, 2003.

54 - Goodson P, Diaz M . Characterizing the adolescent. In: Cavalcanti RC. (Sexual and reproductive health: teaching how to teach. Brasilia: CESEX, 1990. p. 253-268.

55 - Monesi AA. Adolescence and the experience of sexuality. In: Ribeiro M (Org.). Educaçâo sexual: novas ideias, novas conquistas. Rio de Janeiro: Rosa dos Tempos, 1993. p. 91-100.

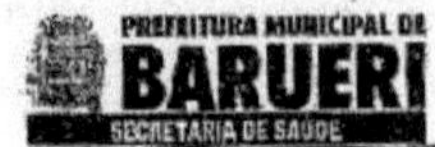

PREFEITURA MUNICIPAL DE BARUERI
SECRETARIA DE SAÚDE

Ofício n.º 1.241/2010
- S. S. -

Barueri, 16 de novembro de 2010

Prezado Secretário,

Solicitamos a Vossa Senhoria autorização para que a Faculdade de Odontologia da Universidade de São Paulo, em parceria com a Secretaria Municipal de Saúde de Barueri, selecionem alguns alunos, entre meninos e meninas, com autorização prévia de seus pais ou responsáveis, a fim de realizar entrevistas complementares relativas ao **Levantamento Epidemiológico das Condições de Saúde Bucal**, ocorrido em outubro de 2009. Segue pedido de autorização anexa.

Contando com a sua colaboração, aproveitamos a oportunidade para renovar os protestos de nossa estima e consideração.

SECRETARIA DE EDUCAÇÃO
Protocolo Geral Nº
Registro no Livro
Entrada em
Encarregado do Protocolo

Atenciosamente,

DR. MAURÍCIO TUNDISI
Secretário de Saúde

Ao
Ilmo. Sr.
CELSO FURLAN
DD. Secretário de Educação
Rua da Prata, nº 727
Jardim dos Camargos – Barueri

RECEBI A 1ª VIA
EM___/___/___

Barueri

Secretaria de Saúde
Rua Prof. João da Matta e Luz, 262 - Centro, Barueri, SP / CEP: 06401-120
Fone: (11) 4199.3100 - e-mail: sameb@sameb.sp.gov.br - www.barueri.sp.gov.br

ANNEX B - Authorization from the school

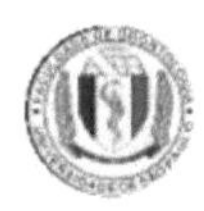

EPIDEMIOLOGICAL SURVEY

OF ORAL HEALTH CONDITIONS

IN THE MUNICIPALITY OF BARUERI,

SAO PAULO, BRAZIL, 2009

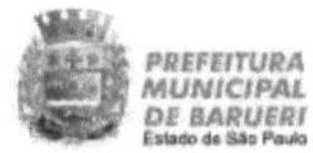

lime. Mr.

Celso Furian

Secretary of Education

Dear Sir,

Please take a few minutes to read this communiqué.

The Faculty of Dentistry of the University of São Paulo, in partnership with the Municipal Health Department of Barueri, carried out a comprehensive survey of oral health conditions in the municipality of Barueri. In this clinical investigation, an interview was carried out to characterize the socio-economic conditions and access to oral health services, and the teeth and gums of children, adolescents, adults and the elderly living in the area covered by the Basic Health Units of the public network were examined.

The examination consisted of an observation of the mouth, carried out in health centers, with all the technique, safety and hygiene, according to the norms of the World Health Organization and the Ministry of Health. There were no risks or discomfort for those who were examined. The individual data will not be divulged under any circumstances, but the results of the research will help a lot to prevent oral diseases and improve everyone's health.

The interviews were carried out with groups of young people, adults and the elderly who attend health centers. However, it will be necessary to carry out new interviews with the group of patients in educational establishments.

We therefore ask for **your understanding and cooperation by authorizing the** participation of the school indicated in the **table below.** We assure you that a group of approximately 20 pupils, including boys and girls, whose parents or guardians have given their prior authorization will be invited to take part in the interview, after receiving the necessary information.

Further information about the work can be obtained from:

Dr. Greice de Brito Souza	Phone: (11) 6398-6647
Prof. Simone Rennó Junqueira	Phone: (11) 3091-7891

Hoping to count on your support, we thank you in advance on behalf of all those who are committed to improving public health in our state and in Brazil.

Sincerely,

Research Coordination

AUTHORIZATION

After being informed about the characteristics of the research "Epidemiological survey of oral health conditions

in the municipality of Barueri, Sâo Pauio, Brazil, 2009", **I AGREE** to the participation of the teaching unit

: EMF MARIO JOAQUIM ESCOBAR DE ANDRADE.

Emde of 20   .

Name of Responsible PersonSignature of Responsible Person

ANNEX C - Approval of CEP

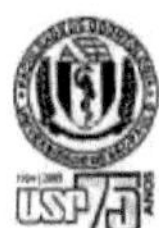

Universidade de São Paulo

Faculdade de Odontologia

Comitê de Ética em Pesquisa

PARECER DE APROVAÇÃO
FR   268264
Protocolo 93/2009

Com base em parecer de relator, o Comitê de Ética em Pesquisa **APROVOU** o protocolo de pesquisa **"Levantamento epidemiológico das condições de saúde bucal no município de Barueri, São Paulo, Brasil, 2009"**, de responsabilidade do Prof.(a) Dr.(a) Antônio Carlos Frias.

Tendo em vista a legislação vigente, devem ser encaminhados a este Comitê relatórios anuais referentes ao andamento da pesquisa e ao término cópia do trabalho em "cd". Qualquer emenda do projeto original deve ser apresentada a este CEP para apreciação, de forma clara e sucinta, identificando a parte do protocolo a ser modificada e suas justificativas.

São Paulo, 10 de agosto de 2009.

Prof. Dr. João Gualberto de Cerqueira Luz
Coordenador do CEP-FOUSP

ANNEX D - Informed Consent Form

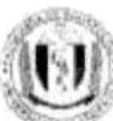 LEVANTAMENTO EPIDEMIOLÓGICO DAS
CONDIÇÕES DE SAÚDE BUCAL NO MUNICÍPIO DE
BARUERI, SÃO PAULO, BRASIL, 2009 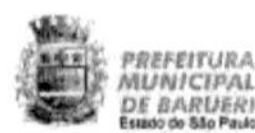

Termos de Consentimento Livre e Esclarecido

São Paulo, outubro de 2009.

Prezado Senhor

Pedimos o favor de dedicar alguns minutos do seu tempo para ler este comunicado.

A Faculdade de Odontologia da Universidade de São Paulo, em parceria com Secretaria Municipal de Saúde de Barueri, realizarão um Levantamento Epidemiológico das Condições de Saúde Bucal, no município de Barueri. Nessa investigação científica, será realizada uma entrevista para caracterização das condições sócio-econômicas e de acesso aos serviços de saúde bucal e serão examinados os dentes e as gengivas de adultos e idosos residentes na área de abrangência de Unidades Básicas de Saúde da rede pública. O exame é uma observação da boca, com toda técnica, segurança e higiene, conforme normas da Organização Mundial da Saúde e do Ministério da Saúde.

Para tanto, o(a) senhor(a) está sendo **convidado(a)** para participar desta pesquisa de forma totalmente voluntária. Não representa riscos nem desconforto para quem será examinado. Os dados individuais não serão divulgados em nenhuma hipótese, mas os resultados da pesquisa ajudarão muito a prevenir doenças bucais e melhorar a saúde de todos.

Antes de concordar em participar desta pesquisa e responder à entrevista é muito importante que o (a) senhor(a) compreenda as informações contidas neste documento. As equipes de pesquisa poderão responder todas as suas dúvidas antes que decida se quer participar. Em qualquer momento da pesquisa ou da entrevista o(a) Sr(a) poderá retirar o consentimento sem qualquer prejuízo. Por isso, **sua colaboração, autorizando no quadro abaixo a realização do exame**, é muito importante.

Esperando contar com seu apoio, desde já agradecemos em nome de todos os que se empenham para melhorar a saúde pública em nosso Estado e no Brasil.

AUTORIZAÇÃO

Após ter sido informado sobre as características da pesquisa "LEVANTAMENTO EPIDEMIOLÓGICO DAS CONDIÇÕES DE SAÚDE BUCAL NO MUNICÍPIO DE BARUERI, SP, BRASIL, 2009" **AUTORIZO** a realização do exame em:

Nome: ____

Em _____ de _____________________ de 2009.

____
Assinatura do Responsável

Se quiser mais informações sobre o trabalho, por favor ligue para:
Faculdade de Odontologia USP – Dep. Odontologia Social – fone 3091-7891
Secretaria Municipal de Saúde do município de Barueri – fone 4199-3100 ramal 3267

Atenciosamente,

Prof. Dr. Antônio Carlos Frias　　**Dr. Alberto Luiz Kesslering**
Coordenador da Pesquisa　　*Coordenador de Saúde Bucal de Barueri*

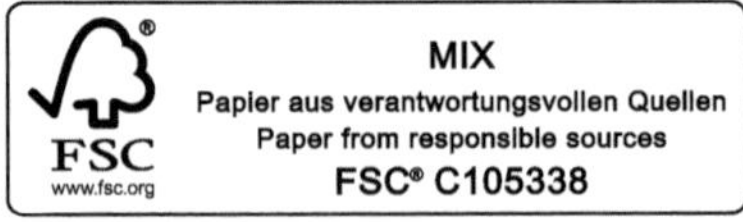

Printed by Books on Demand GmbH, Norderstedt / Germany